My
Champions

Janice Milligan Anderson

Janice Milligan Anderson

ISBN:1499381379
ISBN-13:9781499381375

DEDICATION

In Memory of

My-Daughter-in-Law

Lynn Howell Anderson

My Brother

James C Milligan, Jr

My Sisters

Betty (Tico) Milligan Gibbs

Jane (Sally Jane) Milligan Berger

My Cousin

Charlene Matlock Crawford

Special Thanks to

My Mentor

Dr. Paul E. Cundey, Jr., MD

and

Dr. Kraig Wangsnes, MD

Dr. Mike Holman, MD

Dr. Jeremiah Wilson, MD

Cardiac Cath Lab Teams

Cardiac Rehabilitation Program

Nursing Staff – Heart Tower

at

University Hospital

Augusta, Georgia

Salvation Army, Kroc Center

Augusta, Georgia

CONTENTS

People

According to a source, the song "People", by Jule Styne and Bob Merrill was written in approximately thirty minutes. I have to wonder how such an incredible melody came to light in such a brief period of time.

People, people who need people, are the luckiest people in the world. Interesting, isn't it, that we all know that, but we hardly take the time to acknowledge we depend on others, we need others and that we learn from others.

I for one, am grateful that I had the opportunity to learn the incredible resilience of human courage and survival. May I be a beacon of light for those following me.

The people that were a guiding light for me were real. Most of the time, now, I look and listen to people very differently. I try to absorb the gift of emotional energy they radiate.

The time was difficult for me. I had never been knocked off my pedestal. When I found myself in the position of depending on others for my care, physically and emotionally, I felt insulted yet grateful at the same time. People, people need people. Little did I know there would be people hiding in the future ready to set an example for me. I hope I have learned to be more humble and appreciative of recuperative powers. And, so, I march forward, seeking and learning what is important in life. For sure, there is something I know to be true, people need people.

My Name is Ms Maintenance

Now that is a silly name. I chose this name because I thought it was appropriate for the story and message. Actually, my name is Janice/Jan/Queen and maybe some I don't know about.

The name, Maintenance, right now, suits me well, because I'm just trying to maintain a level of physical activity. In my past, I'm sure there are physical therapists that would laugh and be amazed that I had made it this far. I've said it before and here it goes again - I hate sweating, messing up my hair and please don't ask me to get my hands dirty.

As I progressed through the phases of physical rehabilitation I met some extraordinary people. These people had no idea that they were making such an impact on my recovery efforts. This is why I also named myself Ms Peepers. I watched others. I am aware that staff played an important role, but it was the people in similar and worst circumstances than myself that brought me forward and set the example for me. If there is such a thing as reincarnation, I want to come back as a mega research pharmaceutical scientist so that I can invent an exercise pill. That way I don't have to sweat, I don't have to worry about my hair and I don't have to have a special wardrobe that I can't wear shopping.

And so I travel on to a new exercise regime. I wanted to be livelier and have some choices in my activities. So I tried Tai Chi, Zumba, Water Aerobics and continued with the blessed treadmill. Please excuse me, I have to rest now.

I want to introduce you to a few people. People that had no idea they were looking at an exercise dropout. These people gave my battery a charge so that I could continue this journey. Bless all of you. May I inspire someone as you have inspired me.

Bob

Several times I had noticed him walking the treadmill. I was extremely proud that I was walking 15 minutes on the treadmill at a slow pace. Here he was at a brisk pace. Yep, that is where I want to be one day, on that exercise device, trotting along.

One of my first days of unmonitored exercise, he approached me. "Hello, my name is Bob". "Hello Bob, My name is Janice". I suppose one could say that he became one of my cheerleaders. His advice was simple but I had difficulty with it, "slow it down, be patient, keep at it, it will come". I wanted to push, push, and get it done faster. I wanted to trot on that contraption just like he did.

Then one day he asked me a question - "What are you doing here"? So, I told him my story. Then, I had to ask, "What are you doing here"? At first I wanted to hide in shame. My journey had been nothing compared to what his must have been. Then my next thoughts were, okay, if he can do this under those circumstances, I can do it. Three times a week his comments were generally "slow it down, or you're doing great, build on this exercise plan slowly, otherwise you'll hurt yourself".

Oh, his reason for being in rehab; two years prior to my meeting him, double lung transplant. The man could walk the treadmill a minimum of 45 minutes at a moderate pace. He claims that the reason for his success was that he was in exercise rehab before the transplant.

Barbara

"Hello, my name is Barbara". That is how our conversation began.

During my early course of physical rehab I had noticed a slender lady come in, go to a closet, take out a long green oxygen tube. She would then walk over to the oxygen delivery column, connect the tubing and then climb aboard a treadmill. It seemed to me that she would walk and walk. I also noticed that despite her long green tubing she could actually walk and talk at the same time. Various patients and staff would go stand by the treadmill and talk while she walked. Yep, I want to be that way when I am promoted to another level.

It happened one day that we walked side by side. We exchanged a greeting that first day, occasionally would smile, but that was the only communication we had that day.

Our visits to rehab coincided and we began to forward march on the treadmill, frequently side by side . One day she asked why I was there. I diluted the story and told her. I then asked why she was there. The lady look healthy except for the long green tubing. When she told me her story I was so glad that I had diluted my story. Her story was amazing. She had a Mercer (MRSA) Staff Infection in her right lung. During her hospital stay she had respiratory arrest 3 times. Interesting to me was that she had been physically active when that happened to her. I hate exercise, but this information does speak to me.

The lady is walking and talking while utilizing the mechanics of the treadmill. In the meantime while trying to maneuver on this blasted thing, my tongue is hanging out and I might need oxygen.

Cindy

There she was at the center of Zumba class. Exercise attire and wireless microphone on. Ready? Ready? Music playing, now dance. Dance, don't stand there with your mouth open, move it. She didn't say that, but I thought it.

No clue what was happening, but I moved - in the wrong direction. The lady next to me laughed and told me it was okay, just move, I'd learn the steps. So, I moved, occasionally up against the wall. Gee-whiz, don't know if I can survive this.

Finally after 30 minutes of shaking my booty, turning around, moving my arms, performing squats and other uninhibited maneuvers, I struggled to a bench and watched body torture for the next 30 minutes. I watched people; it was infectious. They laughed, they moved and it was not a synchronized exhibit. I want to do this!

These people were having such a great

time and Cindy, the instructor was spreading the joy. Cindy could make you laugh. She had a unique way of clapping while moving and looking at her class and saying, "Oh, Yes, let's move it". After class I went up to Cindy, apologized for sitting out the last half of the class. I briefly explained my inability to perform Broadway style. She gave me a little hug then said, "Honey, just keep at it. You should have seen me when I first started, pitiful". In the year 2011 she was in a wheelchair. This year is 2013 and she is now a certified Zumba instructor.

I want what she's got, but I have to work at it. There is no magic potion.

Connie

We weren't buddies, rather long time acquaintances. Both of us were in the same profession, shared other friendships and had a mutual respect going on. I had a sense of pride just knowing her.

By way of our social networking, I learned that she was having some health issues that were similar to mine. Some of the recommended procedures were also similar.

There was a long conversation between the two of us. I knew about her close family losses, but, I never knew about some of the obstacles she had over come. There was a shoulder replacement, hip replacement, other surgeries and now other symptoms creeping in. But there was that **SMILE**, radiant, kind, but stay out of my way if something is amiss.

I had a deep sense of concern about her surgery and recovery. The woman all but leaped off the recovery bed. No, things did not go perfectly, but her ability to push toward recovery and put that smile on her face just made her efforts appear near effortless. Is fortitude genetic, learned or magically deposited at ones doorstep? If it is magic, then please, Merlin, you don't have to ring the doorbell when you leave it there. I'll find it when I walk out the door to exercise.

Labrador

I don't know if it matters, but Labrador is a dog that looks sweet and docile. Somehow I'm trying to imagine what the Lab is thinking, *The woman writing about me doesn't really know me, she just watches me. She can't figure out why my owner has me. I have the usual guide dog harness that is held by my owner.*

Ms Peepers is fascinated by me; she wants to pet me but is hesitant because she doesn't know the rules for Service Dogs.

When my owner is participating in water aerobics, I'm allowed to lie on the floor, on towels, next to the life guard. A plunge might be nice, but I won't do it. I watch my owner and occasionally peek at Ms Peepers, I think, because she stares at me.

It is obvious that Labrador is devoted. Again, mirrored in my mind is the indication that people are becoming more physically active. I hate exercise and I'm waiting on a metamorphosis

turning me into an exercising Queen.
Maybe I need a Lab Doggie to bite me
in the butt when I get slack.

Ms Blond

I didn't know her name. Oh, she told me, but I was so fascinated that I didn't remember. I had seen her several times around the facility and thought that she walked with charm and grace.

And there she was in Zumba class. She was tall and slender and had an incredible body form. Why did I have to be so vertically challenged? She knew the steps and would even call out approval during the routine. It was obvious she wasn't a new kid on the block like yours truly.

Now, she might be tall and slender, but I could be short and slender, couldn't I? *Just work it girl*, I would tell myself as my tongue hung out of my mouth. Move or fall on the floor.

Again, after 30 minutes I sat on the side lines and watched the ending performance. During the cool down

period, someone announced that the
tall blond figure was 74 years old!!
Someone lies, I know they lie .

Ms Knees

I met Ms Knees in the ladies locker room. We exchanged pleasantries. I watched as she rubbed ointment on her knees. I asked if she was in pain. She told me that she stayed in pain, but that she was much better. Being curious, or nosy, your call on that one, I asked why she was in pain. She explains it all to me. I just sat on the bench, startled look on my face, my mouth slightly opened as I listened to the story. As she spoke, she placed some articles across her walker. She had been in the pool and that helped her knees.

Bone on bone was her explanation of the pain in her knees. She had been over weight, couldn't have surgery and the water was a helpful relief. Plus it helped her move her legs better.

At some point in time, Ms Knees, decided that she had to get some of that weight off. She had to keep those legs moving. OMG! OMG! Yes, she did, she got on the treadmill. For over a year, this soul has walked the treadmill, **EVERY DAY,** has lost over 40 pounds and the knees that were once surrounded by fat, now have creases. "Oh, yes, it still hurts, but I've made such progress", was her comment. You don't find strength under a rock, you find it with gut wrenching determination. I'm still looking for mine.

No Name Lady

I never talked to her. As she passed me I would occasionally whisper to her "Good Job" and that sweet smile would appear on her face.

I had watched her progress as she struggled to walk the track, first with a walker, next without the walker but with assistance and finally alone. Her right foot would drag. But she did it.

I wondered if she was as proud of herself as I was proud of her. I had the feeling that she sensed my approval. She always had that smile when we looked at each other.

I never really knew her story, but sensed it was one painful emotional bang. But here she was, determined. Actually I felt insignificant in her presence. I say that simply because I imagined her struggles had been more significant than mine. Our thoughts were probably the same, *If she can do it, I can do it.*

The day that she first walked the treadmill was horrifying for me. I was prepared to jump and catch her when she fell. Silly woman, ME. She didn't fall, she smiled, I breathed easier and watched her perform that task. I smiled and whispered, "Good Job".

Sarah and John

"Hello, my name is Sarah. The man over there is John, he's my husband, he's 90 years old and I'm 83. You're new here, aren't you"? I was getting ready to start the treadmill and she had climbed aboard the machine next to me. Our conversation began before the blasted machines could be fired up.

I told her the level I was in the program and that I had been here for a number of weeks. She informed me that they had to travel many miles to get to the rehab gym. They had tried other facilities but only saw unfriendly young people there. The couple decided that distance made no difference and they would make the trek. So here I stand before this couple, waiting and watching. Yes, they did! They hit the start button on the contraptions and walked and walked. She talked and talked, he smiled and smiled.

Usually I listen to my iPod with upbeat music when I walked. But she talked, so I listened. I watched closely, she could breath

while walking. She walked while talking, for
3/4 mile. I did find out that we had one thing
in common - we both hated exercise. Ninety
year old husband walked about 3/4 mile and
then went on to other workout equipment.
He's 90 and has good-looking legs.

Shuffling Man

Each day that I went to exercise I had goals. First and foremost, get it done. The second goal, get the first treadmill in that long line of walking/running machines. You see, the first treadmill gave me visual access into the pool room and the entry door into all of the exercise equipment and rooms. It was like I was my own spy-cam.

There I was, one day, walking along on the lead demon, when a gentleman enters the exercise area. By now I have realized that it is ridiculous to try guessing anyone's age. I watched as he slowly walked down the corridor in front of me. I was preparing myself to jump off my magical walking broomstick to lend a fellow human a hand. Again, silly me. Shortly the gentleman emerged in the pool room and then got in the pool. He bounced around a little in the water, and then he would swim laps.

I am suffering here from *why can't
I do that Syndrome.* One of the first
lessons that I have learned is get off
your BUTT and eat your Wheaties .

Tiny Lady

I'm trying to make a decision. I need to pick an exercise routine that I will stick with. You already have the idea now that I am not an exercise buff. So, I really need to find things that I like and that should help me with my problem of being physically lazy.

I tried Tai Chi. Yes, I liked this, but the instructor was a gentle soul and I couldn't hear him. However, I did notice this tiny woman in front of me and I tried to follow her movements. I did a miserable job, but it is something I think I would like. If only I could hear the quiet instructions and knew the maneuvers. So, I watched the little lady move and tried to follow her. I truly think this is the time in my life that I fully realized that I was a klutz. The men in that class exhibited far more graceful moves than I could manage.

So, let's proceed to Zumba Class. Hoot-hoot. This is loud and my kind of venue - maybe.

Tiny woman is also in Zumba class. Her

movements in Tai Chi were so proficient. I felt it safe to assume that Zumba was merely a trial thing for her. WRONG! This little lady could move it. Here again, she was in front of me, but at this pace there was no following anyone for me.

I cannot make it through an hour's worth of Zumba. Thirty minutes, right now, is my limit and that is accompanied by several wall leanings.

My other new heroine - Little Lady, well, she is 80 years old. Oh, before I forget, Little Lady also does Yoga. Imagine that. I'm doomed.

Yolanda

The first time that I met her she was connecting me to a monitor. You've had the feeling before, you meet someone and there is just an unexplained alliance. Nurse Yolanda did that for me. She didn't bring out pom-poms but I could sense that she was on my team. Each day I waited on her approving smile and I got it.

Then one day she said to me, "You know, you're doing amazingly well. We're very proud for you". Yolanda didn't know that she had just handed me a trophy sticker that read *I'm Inspiring.* If I had been acting, I'm sure I could have won an Academy Award. But I wasn't acting; I was performing for my life.

After that, my imagination went wild. I could just envision myself, on the treadmill, loping along at a rapid pace, raising my arms in the air and yelling,

Hey, Nurse Yolanda, look no hands.
At that point I'm sure I would have
fallen backwards off the treadmill, and
then rushed to Orthopedics and after
that taken for a mental health
evaluation.

Truthfully, Yolanda did not give me a
performance sticker, only because she
didn't have one. But I got the message,
so now I'll take my bow.

Yes, yes, all Nurse Yolandas out there,
take a bow.

From Where I Stood

Ever since I can remember I wanted to be in Health Care. I chose Nursing. Very early in my career a situation happened that stimulated my curiosity and need for continued serious learning. That led me to a career in Cardiac Nursing. I loved it, cherished it and learned.

Spiked interest had developed in Acute Care for the Cardiac patient in our area. I had the opportunity to join a team that provided cardiovascular monitoring. What a challenge and learning experience. With this forward motion of critical care in our community, my hunger for knowledge provided an opportunity to assimilate medical and patient care in an insulated environment.

It was intriguing to learn more about the functions of the cardiovascular system. But, it was surprising to hear and learn the thought provoking reactions and concerns expressed by the patients and families. Interesting, because at that point in time not much credence was given to this side of patient care. To this day, I remember some of those patients. I remember their names, their families and their stories. Fascinating that some of those young wives went on to become Nurses. I like to think that our team had a positive impact on them.

One Christmas night, I found myself on the receiving end of Critical Care. As I looked back on those days and weeks, I couldn't help but wonder if my actions, in the pioneering days, had meant as much to others as others were now giving to me.

Swing Low Sweet Chariot

That night the Chariot did swing low, but not low enough. It missed me. I might have had a little ride, but there was an interventional physician and staff protecting me and steering the chariot in another direction. Way To Go TEAM.

All of this was new for me. I'd never been critically ill before and I don't want to go there again. But, if I must have the experience again and if you are in-charge, may I please have the same TEAM?

I remember the scurrying, but mostly I remember my very favorite PJ's being cut off. And oh, I remember the gentleness. "We're with you. We are going to take care of you"; . Oh yes, I do remember those words and the touching of my hand.

Wonderful people rendered my care. Most were warm and comforting. I sincerely hope that your great care was my just reward. I tried hard to be a good nurse.

Bogginess

Who ever heard of that word –
Bogginess. It didn't pass the spell
check. If you drive an automobile, I'm
sure at some time you have been stuck
in the mud or something. Remember
how you probably spun the wheels
trying to get out of the stuckidness
(that didn't pass the spell check either,
but I'm leaving it). Spin, spin those
wheels and you go nowhere. So, you
get out and you try to push the thing.
Not much luck, that vehicle is bigger
than you. Soon a passerby approaches,
"Can I help"? Now, what are you
going to do? Are you going to get out
your hand held device and look on
Face book, Twitter or WebMD?

My Point? I'm saying that we have
become so excited and bogged down
by our technology that often we have
forgotten our purpose and goals,
healing and comfort. Understand, I
applaud the technological creations. I

love the computer and though some devices can talk back to me, they are not consistently comforting, nor can they be humble.

What we obtain from technological devices is information. Assimilation of the data isn't always left up to us. Frequently algorithms are provided, indicating if this happens, then do this. Common sense tells you when to act or not react to the suggestions provided by the algorithms. Oh, I know, I know, someone has written something. But it sounds robotic. I ask where is the soul/spirit in the response?

It was PEOPLE that moved me forward. PEOPLE gave me inspiration. PEOPLE gave me smiles. PEOPLE set examples. I watched and like a sponge I soaked up some of your motivation and joy.

Rehab Therapist

I had been in a hospital for almost one month. The exercise area was a large open space area surrounded by windows. Outside looked like a perfectly beautiful day. She did, she did. She took me outside for my activity. Tears came into my eyes, I was outside!!

Another time a Therapist had me dancing, sideways, with her, holding my hands, three steps to the left, then three steps to the right. So much laughter by both of us. At each session, I was encouraged to yank it up a gear. I remember the first time I walked the entire length of the hall. I had this big grin on my face. Another staff member walked by, saw us grinning and promptly announced, "Show off". Rolls of laughter went down that hallway and yes, indeed, I was showing off.

The Home Health Therapist took

me outside every chance she got for my activity. Then she spent extra time looking for activity games I could do with my Wii Console. When I climbed my first set of stairs, she clapped and I got a hug.

Nurses and Therapists in Cardiac Rehab were encouraging, never pushy. All of this made me want to do it, get better.

A Conversation

We laughed about what I thought was my sweating problem, meaning, that I didn't like it. Then we giggled about the exercise clothing. I had to admit that it was comfortable but certainly not charming and fashionable unless you have a magnificent body. Oh well, I lack the fashionable magnificent body .

Before we really got into the whys and importance of aggressive body movements we talked about how we were raised. During our time, our parents let us cut-out paper dolls, play with dolls, play the piano, have tea parties and whatever was considered *ladylike* at the time. Oh, that's it, blame it on the parents. Listen, they didn't know. Personally, I would still like to ignore the benefits of exercise. Right now I'm trying to find some cheap reward system that will help to keep me going.

We certainly agreed that there was an abundance of evidence that supported the beneficial effects of exercise. Now, here is something I need to say: I should never be embarrassed or ashamed to say that I don't like exercise, but I do it because it helps me to at least keep status quo. Oh, I can hear you right now, you exercise buffs; I hear you suck in your deep breath and get prepared for a verbal fight. Just chill, dude or duchess, I don't have to do things YOUR WAY.

As we hung up the phone we both agreed that I was doing the right thing, sweating at the appropriate times - exercise times. Now, I have to go walk the treadmill, perform water aerobics and probably sit in the whirlpool. And, yes, I need to look for more inspirational people. Will you be one of them?

Hokey Pokey

You are probably far to young to recall the old song and dance - *The Hokey Pokey.* The words and dance moves remind me of physical rehabilitation moves. Start slow and build on those moves or exercise routines.

Start with an imaginary circle. *You put your right foot in, you take your right foot out. You put your right foot in and shake it all about.* In the dance you go through all of your main body parts and at the end you jump into the circle, jump out, then jump back in the circle and shake your body. While you are doing all of these gyrations, you are singing the song. Try it! It is funny and silly, but you are moving.

So, why would I mention this silly little exercise song? Listen, if you detest exercise as much as I do, you will use every fun mechanism available to get your booty moving. Another justification for mentioning the *fun* is because of sourpuss Therapists and Trainers. Some are so far into body torture that they have forgotten the fun that will lead to the rewards. Along the way I've met a few of you Master Sergeants: You *ain't* fun and your tactics don't work on me. I say to you, "Get your head out of the clouds, put a smile on your face and work WITH me, don't BOSS me".

Allow me to mention a young man named Zach. Several times he walked me post-operatively. I always looked forward to his visits. I didn't want to walk, it hurt, and it wore me out, but Zach had ways of getting my mind off of the chore by engaging in delightful conversations. He took the time to learn about me. Young man, Blessings for you.

The moral of this story? Those of us in Health Care Delivery have a tendency to be robotic in our responses. We become filled with self importance. Patient's and families sense those negative vibes. Only when it *happens to us* do we then take our own inventory. Ouch, that hurts.

Yesterday and Today

When I was a child I rode the bike, skated on the sidewalk, played volley ball, softball, played hide and seek and chased the other children in the neighborhood. I remember my parents playing basketball in the church league. What happened? How and why did we let ourselves become so sedate. It was like physical activity became socially unacceptable.

Now, later in my life, I'm confronted with the benefits of regular physical activity. I'd like nothing better than to tell you to *stick it in your ear;* you have no proof of the added benefits to my well being. But that would be a lie. I've been the recipient of the rewards. Though the rewards have been accepted and life is more energetic, I still don't like it. But I will persist for the value of living and laughing for a few more years.

I will not be a fanatic about this activity, but I will plaster a smile on my face and proceed through the walk for my life. I don't have an exercise buddy. Some have made that suggestion to me. No, I will not make a competition out of this. I already have a competitor - and my competitor is my LIFE.

The guilt creeps into my mind. I did not set an example for my children. They have the genes. One day those genes will rear up in ugliness.

I perform now - for MY LIFE.

Open My Eyes

Remember the words to the old Hymn *Open My Eyes?* The Hymn starts off with *open my eyes that I might see glimpses of truth.* Truly, I thought that I was aware of my truth and that I was knowledgeable when it came to the health of body and mind. When reality smacked me, I realized that I only knew a small amount about the recovery process. Only when I had to deal with a recovery did I confront the issues of my ignorance of the profound strength that was required to RALLY against the odds.

What I had to do was open my eyes, take off my rose tinted glasses, then watch and listen. Watch the struggle, physically and mentally, by those affected by disease. Listen as they told their stories or just imagining what that story might be. I watched the people walking with canes or walkers. I watched the wheelchairs being ushered in. My problem was insignificant.

All these years, how did I miss the significant wrestling match that others might have. Like others, I'm sure, it was not that I didn't care, but rather, that I was absorbed in other parts of life. The saying of *stop and smell the roses* should remind us that there are other things in life that hold significance for us.

My Champions were everyday people. These people had taken the insult that was hurled at them, made a mockery of the insult and came up a winner in the Lottery of Life. It has been like I was at a buffet filled with life's stories of courage and determination. I can help myself to anything on the buffet, all I have to do is look at the spread before me.

Family Champions

I dedicated this book to members of my family that fought formidable battles with various diseases.

These losses took an emotional toll on the family. It was painful to watch the deterioration of the bodies of our loved ones, but the loss of the soulfulness was shattering.

My family members, Lynn, Jim, Jane, Betty and Charlene, you continue to be loved as though your bodies are still present among us. Memories are embedded, forever, in our hearts and minds.

'Till we meet again.

ABOUT THE AUTHOR

Born and raised in Savannah, Georgia. She moved to Augusta, Georgia to pursue a career in Nursing. Goal accomplished she entered the field of Acute Cardiac Care and was a pioneer in that field for the Augusta area. In addition to Nursing she also added a second track to her career, Cardiac Sonography.

Now retired, she pursues whatever she wants. Also, the Author of <u>Home to Savannah</u>.

www.ingramcontent.com/pod-product-compliance
Lightning Source LLC
Chambersburg PA
CBHW071330310526
45789CB00017B/2173